Low Carb Recipes

50 Vegetarian and Vegan Recipes for Successful Weight Loss in Just 2 Weeks

Mathias Müller

Copyright © 2016 Mathias Müller

All rights reserved.

Images: Fotolia
Copy-Editing, Proofreading: Mathias Müller

Published by:
Mathias Müller
Woltmanstraße 10
20097 Hamburg

ISBN-13: 978-1543144734

ISBN 10: 154314473X

TABLE OF CONTENTS

INTRODUCTION 7
Breakfast Recipes 10
    Fruit Yogurt.. 10
    Almond Pancakes 11
    Scrambled Tofu.. 12
    Avocado-Mint Smoothie 13
    Fruit Salad with Yogurt-Basil Dressing............................... 14
    Bell Pepper Omelet 15
    Apple-Walnut Granola... 16
    Green Smoothie 17
    Scrambled Egg with Feta 18
    Parmesan Fried Eggs... 19
Soups and Salads 20
    Mango Salsa with Feta 20
    Artichoke Salad... 21
    Red Beet Salad.. 22
    Celery Salad 23
    Lamb's Salad with Raspberry Dressing.............................. 24
    Spinach Soup with Fried Egg 25
    Cream of Tomato Soup... 26
    Mixed Cabbage Soup 27
    Carrot Soup with Citrus Fruits 28
    Mushroom Broth 29
Lunch Recipes... 30
    Parsley Root Fries 30
    Green Omelet.. 31
    Zucchini Pasta with Caper Pesto 32
    Mozzarella Mushrooms with Tomato Pesto 33
    Minestrone with Seasonal Vegetables 34

- Vegan Shish Kebabs 35
- Zucchini Carpaccio 36
- Carrot Curry 37
- Kohlrabi Au Gratin 38
- Scalloped Fennel 39

Dinner Recipes 40
- Parmesan-Crusted Celery Scallops 40
- Sage Omelet 41
- Parsnip Stir-Fry 42
- Pumpkin-Mozzarella Casserole 43
- Stuffed Mushrooms 44
- Baked Asparagus 45
- Vegetable Kebabs 46
- Eggplant Lasagna 47
- Stuffed Peppers 48
- Cauliflower Casserole 49

Snacks 51
- Pepper Snack 51
- Spicy Kale Chips 52
- Dolmades 53
- Carrot Patties 54
- Chicory Boats 55
- Pumpkin Chips with Parmesan 56
- Vegetarian Patty 57
- Stuffed Tomatoes 58
- Baked Chèvre 59
- Tofu Patties 60

CONCLUSION 61
AUTHOR 62

INTRODUCTION

Vegetarians and vegans, just like other nutritional styles, often face prejudice. This typically starts with the assumption that a meatless diet and being overweight are generally mutually exclusive. But the many vegetarians and vegans still struggling with their weight show this is not actually the case. This is quite often due to the diet being higher in carbs, which is not good for the metabolism. And yet many vegetarians and vegans find it hard to go low carb, since they're afraid of having to forgo a lot of the ingredients they're familiar with.

My goal in writing this cookbook was therefore to choose recipes which clearly focus on great taste. Since I've encountered so many vegetarians and vegans over my years of practice who found it hard to reconcile their lifestyle with a diet, I found it especially important to leave out the traditional approaches of a diet and instead clearly demonstrate the connection between certain food groups and weight loss. Even those who aren't familiar with the low carb rules will quickly have a good understanding just from cooking. However, the good feeling you will soon have when you start losing the first few pounds, is much more important.

The benefits of the low carb cuisine are that it goes with any generation and any budget. So families will still be able to enjoy the same meal. After all, low carb doesn't mean cutting out carbs completely, but simply reducing the amount. You therefore don't need to worry about nutrient deficiency, since you won't feel hungry or have a shortage of carbs. This helps the body maintain its performance level and you will stay motivated to eat low carb. This can be confirmed by David, a 36-year-old bricklayer:

"I purposely switched to low carb when I had 5 days off so I'd be able to determine how it affects my fitness. After just a few days I already noticed that I wasn't feeling groggy and scatter-brained like with other diets, but actually felt full of energy after every meal. Even during the second week and after a tough day of physical labor at work I still had enough energy at night to keep up with family and friends. "

Showing more confidence in your environment after just two weeks may sound ambitious, but with these recipes you can have that whenever you're ready. After all, in addition to being noticeably overweight, the looks or comments in public often have a much greater impact on your mind. When these negative experiences turn into positive compliments, your confidence will automatically grow. So take this important step to starting a new chapter in your life. This cookbook provides instructions for a healthy diet and will increase your pleasure and quality of life with every meal. Losing weight without abstaining or feeling hungry will allow you to gain new body awareness without having to deviate from your vegetarian or vegan lifestyle.

Breakfast Recipes

Fruit Yogurt

Ingredients for 4 servings:
- 1 1/2 c (400 g) Greek yogurt
- 2/3 c (100 g) blackberries
- 1/3 c (50 g) unsalted cashews
- Agave syrup to sweeten

Directions:
1. Add the yogurt to a bowl and mix in with the washed blackberries.
2. Chop the cashews and add to the yogurt. If you don't want to chop the cashews with a knife, you can also put them in a freezer bag and crush with a pan. To do so, make a layer of nuts in a freezer bag and use the bottom of the pan as a hammer.
3. Lastly sweeten with agave syrup, if you'd like.

Time: 5 minutes
Difficulty: Easy

Nutrition facts per serving:
Calories: 250 kcal
Fat: 9.4 g
Protein: 16.2 g
Carbohydrates 12.2 g

Almond Pancakes

<u>Ingredients for 4 servings:</u>
- 2/3 c (100 g) ground almonds
- 1 c (100 g) protein powder
- 2 Tbs (25 g) sugar substitute, e.g. Stevia or Splenda
- 1 1/2 c (350 ml) milk
- 1 vanilla bean
- 5 tsp (1 pkg) baking powder
- Oil

Directions:
1. In a bowl whisk the ground almonds, protein powder, sugar substitute, baking powder and the milk to a smooth batter. To prevent clumps, you can also use a hand mixer.
2. Cut the vanilla bean in half and scrape out the pulp with a knife. Add to the batter and briefly blend again. Heat a pan with oil on the stove, use a ladle to pour pancakes into the hot pan and cook. Cook the almond pancakes about 2-3 minutes each side until golden brown.
3. The almond pancakes are great both warm and cold and you can easily use the different low carb spreads to vary them.

Time: 20 minutes
Difficulty: Easy

<u>Nutrition facts per serving:</u>
Calories: 310 kcal
Fat: 17.2 g
Protein: 29.3 g
Carbohydrates 7.1 g

Scrambled Tofu

Ingredients for 4 servings:
- 7 oz (200 g) tofu
- 4 eggs
- 1 tomato
- 1 onion
- Oil
- Curry powder
- Salt and pepper to season

Directions:
1. Use a fork to crush the tofu in a bowl. Add the eggs and blend. Season with curry powder and with salt and pepper and set aside for a little while.
2. Chop the onion and the tomatoes and keep in separate bowls.
3. Heat a little oil in a pan and first lightly braise the onions until they start to brown. Then add the chopped tomatoes and sauté for 2 minutes. Add the egg-tofu mixture and continue cooking until all of the egg is firm.
4. Then taste the scrambled eggs again and if necessary season. Then serve the scrambled tofu on plates and enjoy warm.

Time: 10 minutes
Difficulty: Easy

Nutrition facts per serving:
Calories: 162 kcal
Fat: 9 g
Protein: 12.5 g
Carbohydrates 5.5 g

Avocado-Mint Smoothie

Ingredients for 4 servings:
- 1 1/2 c (400 g) Greek yogurt
- 1/2 lb (200 g) avocado
- 10 mint leaves

Directions:
1. Peel the avocados, removing all woody areas with a sharp knife. Chop the flesh and add into a shaker.
2. Add the yogurt and blend into a creamy smoothie on high. Add the mint leaves and blend another 30 seconds.
3. Pour the smoothie into cups and serve promptly. Or refrigerate and enjoy later.

Time: 10 minutes
Difficulty: Easy

Nutrition facts per serving:
Calories: 210 kcal
Fat: 17 g
Protein: 4.3 g
Carbohydrates 8.5 g

Fruit Salad with Yogurt-Basil Dressing

Ingredients for 4 servings:
- 3/4 c (200 g) Greek yogurt
- 1/2 lb (200 g) strawberries
- 2/3 c (100 g) blackberries
- 1 papaya
- 15 basil leaves
- 1 Tbs balsamic vinegar
- Pepper to season

Directions:
1. Cut the strawberries in half, cut the papaya into cubes and add both of these and the blackberries to a bowl. Toss with salad servers.
2. Finely chop the basil and mix with the yogurt and balsamic vinegar. I desired, season to taste with pepper. This goes just as well with fruit as balsamic vinegar.
3. Pour the dressing over the fruit salad. Serve promptly or infuse in the fridge.

Time: 20 minutes
Difficulty: Easy

Nutrition facts per serving:
Calories: 90 kcal
Fat: 5.1 g
Protein: 2.7 g
Carbohydrates 5.1 g

Bell Pepper Omelet

Ingredients for 4 servings:
- 6 eggs
- 4 marinated bell peppers
- 1 garlic clove
- Olive oil
- Salt and pepper to season

Directions:
1. Dice the marinated bell pepper and mince the garlic.
2. Beat the eggs in a bowl and mix with the bell pepper and garlic. Season with salt and pepper.
3. Heat a non-stick pan with a little oil. Coat the bottom of the pan with the egg mixture. Cook until the sides start to set. Turn the omelet and also cook the other side until golden brown. Repeat with the remaining omelets.
4. Then fold the omelets in half and serve promptly.

Time: 20 minutes
Difficulty: Mean

Nutrition facts per serving:
Calories: 170 kcal
Fat: 7.4 g
Protein: 9 g
Carbohydrates 2.6 g

Apple-Walnut Granola

(✓ if use plant based milk)

Ingredients for 4 servings:
- 2 apples
- 1 c (100 g) sliced almonds
- 1/2 c (50 g) chopped walnuts
- 7 Tbs (100 ml) milk
- Cinnamon

Directions:
1. Peel the apples and cut into small pieces or sticks. Add into a bowl. Mix with the sliced almonds and chopped walnuts. Season the granola with a pinch of cinnamon.
2. Add the milk and serve promptly.

Time: 10 minutes
Difficulty: Easy

Nutrition facts per serving:
Calories: 296 kcal
Fat: 22.8 g
Protein: 8 g
Carbohydrates 12.2 g

Green Smoothie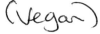

Ingredients for 4 servings:
- 1/2 lb (200 g) fresh spinach
- 1/4 lb (100 g) kale
- 1/4 lb (100 g) rhubarb

Directions:
1. Remove wilted spinach and kale leaves, wash and dry with a salad spinner. Then add the ingredients into a blender.
2. Chop the rhubarb and also add to the blender.
3. Blend into a creamy smoothie on high. Pour into cups or refrigerate.

Time: 10 minutes
Difficulty: Easy

Nutrition facts per serving:
Calories: 19 kcal
Fat: 0.4 g
Protein: 2.5 g
Carbohydrates 1.3 g

Scrambled Egg with Feta

Ingredients for 4 servings:
- 6 eggs
- 1/4 lb (100 g) feta
- 6 cocktail tomatoes
- 1 onion
- Olive oil
- Salt and pepper to season

Directions:
1. Cut the tomatoes in half, peel and cube the onions and keep in separate bowls.
2. Beat the eggs in a bowl and whisk. Then season the egg mixture with salt and pepper.
3. In a pan with a little oil first sauté the onions until slightly light brown. Add the eggs and cook briefly until set. Pull apart the firm eggs.
4. Lastly, add the tomato halves, tear the feta with your hands and also heat in the pan. Sauté another 2 minutes on medium, arrange on plates and serve promptly.

Time: 10 minutes
Difficulty: Easy

Nutrition facts per serving:
Calories: 195 kcal
Fat: 14.5 g
Protein: 13.1 g
Carbohydrates 1.6 g

Parmesan Fried Eggs

Ingredients for 4 servings:
- 4 eggs
- 1 1/2 oz (40 g) Parmesan
- 1 garlic clove
- Oil
- Salt and pepper to season

Directions:
1. Peel and mince the garlic clove. Sauté in a pan with a little oil.
2. Break the eggs into a pan, either all at once or one at a time. Season with salt and pepper. Once the eggs are firm, sprinkle with Parmesan and heat another 30 seconds on medium.
3. Arrange on plates and serve warm. If desired, season with fresh herbs.

Time: 15 minutes
Difficulty: Easy

Nutrition facts per serving:
Calories: 140 kcal
Fat: 10.2 g
Protein: 9.8 g
Carbohydrates 1.4 g

Soups and Salads

Mango Salsa with Feta

Ingredients for 4 servings:
- 1 mango
- 1 cucumber
- 1 green bell pepper
- 1 lime
- 5 oz (150 g) feta
- Olive oil
- Salt and pepper to season

Directions:
1. Peel the cucumber and cut in half lengthwise. Remove the seeds with a teaspoon and dice the flesh. Also dice the mango and add both ingredients into a bowl. Then cut the bell pepper into strips and mix in with the mango and cucumber.
2. Cube the feta and add to the salsa.
3. For the dressing, squeeze the lemon and mix the juice with a little olive oil. Then season the dressing with salt and pepper season and pour over the salad. Toss with salad servers and either serve promptly or refrigerate until ready to serve to enhance flavors.

Time: 10 minutes
Difficulty: Easy

Nutrition facts per serving:
Calories: 169 kcal
Fat: 10.3 g

Protein: 7.5 g
Carbohydrates 10.1 g

Artichoke Salad

Ingredients for 4 servings:
- 1 can artichoke hearts
- 1 yellow bell pepper
- 1 red onion
- ½ bunch of parsley
- 3 1/2 oz (100 g) mozzarella
- White balsamic vinegar
- Olive oil
- Salt and pepper to season

Directions:
1. Peel and dice the red onion. Drain the artichoke hearts in a bowl. Dice the bell pepper.
2. Heat a pan with a little oil and first sauté the onions. Then add the artichokes and bell pepper and heat on medium for 5 minutes.
3. Meanwhile prepare the dressing, mixing equal parts of vinegar and oil. Mix in the chopped parsley and season to taste with salt and pepper.
4. Add the warm vegetables to a bowl with the crumbled or sliced mozzarella and toss with the dressing. Serve warm to bring out the flavors even better.

Time: 10 minutes
Difficulty: Easy

Nutrition facts per serving:
Calories: 117 kcal
Fat: 7.6 g
Protein: 6.2 g
Carbohydrates 4.9 g

Red Beet Salad

Ingredients for 4 servings:
- 1/2 lb (200 g) fresh red beets
- 1/2 lb (200 g) radicchio
- 1 avocado
- 1 lemon
- Olive oil
- Salt and pepper to season

Directions:

1. Cook the red beets in a pot on the stove for about 15 minutes. Do not peel the red beets and if desired add a little salt to the water. Put the red beets on a plate and let cool a bit. Peel and slice or dice with a sharp knife. Here it's best to use disposable gloves so your hands won't stain. Red beets are also available precooked and canned. This will make preparation easier and reduce the overall cooking time.
2. Cut or pluck the radicchio into pieces, wash and dry with a salad spinner. Remove the flesh from the avocado and dice, grate the lemon zest and squeeze the lemon.
3. Add the red beets, lettuce, lemon zest and avocado to a bowl and mix well.
4. For the dressing mix the lemon juice with olive oil, then season with salt and pepper. Pour the dressing over the salad and toss with salad servers. Then serve promptly.

Time: 30 minutes
Difficulty: Mean

Nutrition facts per serving:
Calories: 159 kcal
Fat: 11 g
Protein: 2.8 g
Carbohydrates 10.8 g

Celery Salad

Ingredients for 4 servings:
- 1/2 lb (200 g) celery
- 1/4 lb (100 g) tomatoes on the vine
- 1/2 c (150 g) Greek yogurt
- 2 green onions
- 1 chicory
- 1 garlic clove
- 1 any frozen mixed herbs
- Olive oil
- Salt and pepper to season

Directions:
1. Thinly slice the celery and the green onions and add into a bowl. Quarter the tomatoes and also add into the bowl.
2. Mince the garlic and fry in a pan with a little oil. Cut the chicory in half, season with salt and pepper and sauté on the cut face for about 2-3 minutes. This roasted flavor will add an interesting note to the salad. Remove the lettuce from the pan, cut into strips and mix in with the vegetables in the bowl. Also remove the garlic from the pan and mix in.
3. For the dressing season the yogurt with a few splashes of olive oil and the herbs. Mix the dressing and season to taste with a little salt and pepper. Then either pour the dressing over the salad or pour into a little bowl so everybody can use their preferred amount.

Time: 15 minutes
Difficulty: Easy

Nutrition facts per serving:
Calories: 96.6 kcal
Fat: 6.3 g
Protein: 2.7 g
Carbohydrates 5.9 g

Lamb's Salad with Raspberry Dressing

Ingredients for 4 servings:
- 1/2 lb (200 g) lamb's lettuce
- 1/4 lb (100 g) mozzarella balls
- 2 peaches
- Raspberry dressing
- Oil
- Salt and pepper to season

Directions:
1. Remove the wilted leaves from the lamb's lettuce. Then wash the lettuce and dry with a salad spinner. If the lettuce has a lot of dirt on it, repeat this step.
2. Cut the peaches in half, remove the pit and cut the flesh into wedges with a sharp knife. Season with a little fresh ground pepper and mix with the lettuce and the mozzarella balls in a bowl.
3. For the dressing mix equal parts of raspberry vinegar and oil, and if desired season with salt, pepper or other seasons and fresh herbs.
4. Pour the dressing over the salad and serve promptly.

Time: 10 minutes
Difficulty: Easy

Nutrition facts per serving:
Calories: 122 kcal
Fat: 7.7 g
Protein: 6.2 g
Carbohydrates 6.1 g

Spinach Soup with Fried Egg

<u>Ingredients for 4 servings:</u>
- 1 lb (500 g) fresh spinach
- 2 c (500 ml) vegetable broth
- 1 c (250 ml) coconut milk
- 4 eggs
- 2 onions
- 1 garlic clove
- Oil
- Salt and pepper to season

Directions:
1. Remove wilted leaves of spinach. Place the rest of the spinach in a colander and wash under running water, then dry with a salad spanner. Then chop the spinach with a knife. Next peel and finely dice the onion and mince the garlic.
2. In a pot first lightly braise the garlic and the onions in a little oil on high. It's okay if the onions turns a little brown but not black. Now add the spinach and also lightly braise for about 2 minutes.
3. Add vegetable broth and coconut milk and simmer for about 10 minutes. After this time remove the pot from the burner and slowly puree with an immersion blender. Heat the soup again on medium, and season to taste with salt and pepper.
4. Just before the food is done cooking, cook the eggs sunny side up. Heat a little oil in a pan and either break all eggs in it at once or one at a time and cook. Season with salt and pepper.
5. Pour the soup into soup plates or a small bowl, top with the eggs and serve promptly.

Time: 30 minutes
Difficulty: Easy

<u>Nutrition facts per serving:</u>
Calories: 138 kcal
Fat: 8 g

Protein: 9.6 g
Carbohydrates 6 g

Cream of Tomato Soup

Ingredients for 4 servings:
- 1 large can of tomatoes
- 1 2/3 c (400 ml) vegetable broth
- 1 c (250 g) yogurt
- 1 oz (30 g) ginger
- 1 Spanish onion
- Oil
- Salt and pepper to season

Directions:
1. Peel and dice the Spanish onion and ginger. Lightly braise in a pot with a little oil until translucent. Then add the can of tomatoes. Add the vegetable broth. Bring to a boil, then simmer on medium for 15 minutes.
2. Briefly remove the pot from the burner and puree with an immersion blender. If the tomato soup is too thin, you can add some tomato paste to thicken it up. Reheat the soup and stir in the yogurt a little at a time.
3. Season to taste with salt and pepper and serve on plates or in a tureen. If desired, garnish with fresh herbs, e.g. basil.

Time: 30 minutes
Difficulty: Easy

Nutrition facts per serving:
Calories: 125 kcal
Fat: 9 g
Protein: 3.2 g
Carbohydrates 6.7 g

Mixed Cabbage Soup *Vegan*

<u>Ingredients for 4 servings:</u>
- 1/2 lb (250 g) Brussels sprouts
- 1/2 lb (250 g) broccoli
- 1/2 lb (250 g) Romanesco
- 1 onion
- 1 any frozen mixed herbs
- 6 c (1.5 Liter) vegetable broth
- Oil
- Salt and pepper to season

Directions:
1. First prepare the vegetables, cutting the broccoli and Romanesco into florets and remove the wilted leaves from the Brussels sprouts. Then peel and dice the onion.
2. Heat a pot with oil on the stove and heat the onions in it. They should turn a little brown, but don't burn them. Then add the vegetable broth. Once the broth is hot, add the three vegetables and bring to a boil in the vegetable broth. Then simmer on medium for at least 30 minutes.
3. Season to taste with salt and pepper just before it is done cooking and serve warm.

Time: 40 minutes
Difficulty: Easy

<u>Nutrition facts per serving:</u>
Calories: 83 kcal
Fat: 3 g
Protein: 7.2 g
Carbohydrates 6.1 g

Carrot Soup with Citrus Fruits

Ingredients for 4 servings:
- 1/2 lb (250 g) carrots
- 2/3 c (150 g) crème fraîche
- 2 c (500 ml) vegetable broth
- 1 grapefruit
- 1 Spanish onion
- Oil
- Salt and pepper

Directions:
1. First peel the carrots, then first cut in half and chop. Then peel and dice the onions.
2. Heat a pot with a little oil on the stove and lightly braise the onions until they start to turn colors. Add the diced carrots and heat for 2 minutes, stirring constantly. Add the vegetable broth and bring to a boil. Then cook on medium for 20 minutes. Remove the pot from the burner and puree the soup with an immersion blender. Heat on the stove again, stir in the crème fraîche and season to taste with salt and pepper.
3. Meanwhile prepare the grapefruit sections. First peel the grapefruit. Remove as much of the white skin as possible. With a sharp knife cut along the inner skins and remove the sections of fruit. Keep in a bowl.
4. Serve the soup and garnish with the fruit sections. If desired, add fresh herbs, e.g. chervil or basil to add more flavor.

Time: 30 minutes
Difficulty: Mean

Nutrition facts per serving:
Calories: 188 kcal
Fat: 14 g
Protein: 2.2 g
Carbohydrates 11.3 g

Mushroom Broth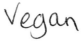

Ingredients for 4 servings:
- 8 oz (200 g) baby mushrooms
- 8 oz (200 g) king oyster mushrooms
- 2 1/2 oz (75 g) celery
- ½ bunch green onions
- 3 1/2 c (750 ml) vegetable broth
- Oil
- Salt and pepper to season

Directions:
1. Slice the mushrooms and lightly braise from both sides in a pan with a little oil to brown. Add into a bowl and set aside.
2. Slice the onions and celery. Heat a pot with oil on the stove and first lightly braise the green onions. They should only be translucent but not turn color. Add the celery and heat 2 more minutes. Add the vegetable broth and heat briefly.
3. Reduce to medium and add the mushrooms. Simmer the soup for 10 more minutes and season to taste with salt and pepper before serving. For an Asian touch you can also add lemongrass, cilantro and chili to the soup.

Time: 20 minutes
Difficulty: Easy

Nutrition facts per serving:
Calories: 50 kcal
Fat: 3 g
Protein: 3.1 g
Carbohydrates 2.6 g

Lunch Recipes

Parsley Root Fries

<u>Ingredients for 4 servings:</u>
- 1 lb (400 g) parsley root
- Paprika
- Oil
- Salt and pepper to season

Directions:
1. Peel the parsley root and cut lengthwise into fries.
2. In a bowl season 2 Tbs olive oil with paprika and salt and pepper. Mix with a whisk or a fork. Add the cut parsley roots and mix well to coat the vegetables with the seasons.
3. Line a cookie sheet with parchment paper and arrange the individual fries on it in a single layer. Bake in a preheated oven at 350°F (180°C) for 20-25 minutes. The cooking time depends on how thick they are cut. Always enjoy the parsley root fries warm for the best taste.

Time: 30 minutes
Difficulty: Easy

<u>Nutrition facts per serving:</u>
Calories: 62 kcal
Fat: 3 g
Protein: 3 g
Carbohydrates 5.4 g

Green Omelet

Ingredients for 4 servings:
- 1/4 lb (100 g) spinach
- 4 eggs
- 2 green onions
- Oil
- Salt and pepper to season

Directions:
1. Thinly slice the green onions. Add into a bowl and set aside for a little while. Then remove the wilted spinach leaves, wash the rest of the spinach and dry in a salad spinner.
2. In a separate bowl beat the eggs with salt and pepper. Then add the eggs and the spinach to a blender and blend on high for about 1 minute.
3. Heat a pan with oil on the stove and first lightly braise the green onions in it. Once they have taken a little color add the egg and spinach mixture. Flip when the edges of the omelet are firm. The remaining cooking time is about half as long as the first side.
4. Arrange on a plate and fold in half before serving. This dish is perfect for invitations, since you can easily make the salmon-cream cheese spread for non-vegetarian guests, which goes perfectly with the spinach flavor.

Time: 20 minutes
Difficulty: Easy

Nutrition facts per serving:
Calories: 404 kcal
Fat: 7.4 g
Protein: 6.5 g
Carbohydrates 2.1 g

Zucchini Pasta with Caper Pesto

Ingredients for 4 servings:
- 2 zucchini
- 1 garlic clove
- 2 oz (50 g) arugula
- 2 oz (50 g) Parmesan
- 2 Tbs (20 g) capers
- Oil
- Salt and pepper to season

Directions:
1. First prepare the pesto. Peel and mince the garlic clove. Add arugula, capers, Parmesan and a little oil to a shaker to make a creamy pesto. Start with just a little oil and add more if necessary. If desired, season the pesto with salt and pepper to taste and refrigerate to infuse until ready to serve.
2. Next wash the zucchini and peel with a vegetable peeler. The shape of the vegetable pasta should be similar to fettuccine.
3. Heat a pan with oil on the stove and lightly braise the zucchini strips for about 3-4 minutes. Divide the zucchini pasta on plates and garnish with dollops of pesto.

Time: 25 minutes
Difficulty: Easy

Nutrition facts per serving:
Calories: 99 kcal
Fat: 6.5 g
Protein: 6.3 g
Carbohydrates 2.9 g

Mozzarella Mushrooms with Tomato Pesto

Ingredients for 4 servings:
- 8 white mushrooms
- 8 mozzarella balls
- 1 1/3 c (75 g) sun-dried tomatoes
- 1 1/2 oz (40 g) Parmesan
- 3/4 c (20 g) basil
- Olive oil
- Salt and pepper to season

Directions:
1. First use a small brush to remove any soil from the white mushrooms. You can also use a new, soft toothbrush for this. Be careful not to apply too much pressure so you won't damage the delicate flesh. Then carefully remove the stems from the white mushrooms and place the white mushrooms on a cookie sheet lined with parchment paper.
2. Then first prepare the pesto for the stuffing. Blend the sun-dried tomatoes and basil, Parmesan and olive oil into a pesto. Start with just a little bit of olive oil and add more as needed.
3. Stuff the white mushrooms with the pesto and add a mozzarella ball to each stuffing. Then bake in a preheated oven at 350°F (180°C) for 20 minutes and serve the stuffed mushrooms warm.

Time: 35 minutes
Difficulty: Easy

Nutrition facts per serving:
Calories: 190 kcal
Fat: 14.1 g
Protein: 11.1 g
Carbohydrates 3.8 g

Minestrone with Seasonal Vegetables

Ingredients for 4 servings:
- 1/4 lb (100 g) green asparagus
- 1/4 lb (100 g) sugar snap peas
- 7 oz (200 g) tofu
- 1 carrot
- 4 1/4 c (1 liter) vegetable broth
- 2 tomatoes
- ½ bunch green onions
- Fresh herbs of your choice to garnish
- Oil
- Salt and pepper to season

Directions:
1. First prepare the vegetables, cutting the woody ends off the green asparagus, and then cut into about 1 1/2 inch (4 cm) pieces. Then peel and slice the carrots. Slice the green onions and sort out the sugar snap peas.
2. Heat a little oil in a pot and first sauté the green onions in it until the white stems are slightly translucent. Add the vegetable broth and bring to a boil. Reduce the heat to medium and first add the sliced carrots and cook for about 5 minutes.
3. Meanwhile chop the tomato and add to the soup along with the cut asparagus and the sugar snap peas. Simmer with the cubed tofu on medium for 15-20 more minutes and season to taste with salt and pepper before serving. The various colors make this minestrone look great in a tureen and guests will also enjoy it. Of course you can also use different seasonal vegetables.

Time: 30 minutes
Difficulty: Easy

Nutrition facts per serving:
Calories: 120 kcal
Fat: 7.4 g

Protein: 6.4 g
Carbohydrates 5.9 g

Vegan Shish Kebabs

Ingredients for 4 servings:
- 1 yellow bell pepper
- 1 green bell pepper
- 1 zucchini
- 2 red onions
- 5 oz (150 g) tofu
- Oil
- Curry powder
- Paprika
- Salt and pepper to season

Directions:
1. First prepare the vegetables, cutting the bell peppers into roughly same size pieces. Also cut the zucchini into bite size pieces and chop the tofu. As a last step peel and quarter the red onions.
2. Thread the vegetables onto wooden skewers, alternating between vegetables, and season with a mix of paprika, curry powder and salt and pepper.
3. Heat a pan with oil on the stove and cook the kebabs on all sides. Of course you can also grill the kebabs. Place on a plate and serve warm.

Time: 20 minutes
Difficulty: Easy

Nutrition facts per serving:
Calories: 97 kcal
Fat: 6.9 g
Protein: 4.4 g
Carbohydrates 2.3 g

Zucchini Carpaccio

Ingredients for 4 servings:
- 2 zucchini
- 1 red onion
- 1 Tbs mustard
- Sherry vinegar
- Oil
- Salt and pepper to season

Directions:
1. To prepare the zucchini, first wash, then thinly slice. Season with salt and pepper in a bowl and toss well.
2. Heat a pan with oil on the stove and sauté the seasoned zucchini slices golden brown from both sides.
3. Arrange the zucchini on plates or a platter. To make the dressing, first dice the red onion. In a small bowl mix equal parts of sherry vinegar and oil. Stir in 1 tsp mustard and the diced onion. Season to taste with salt and pepper, drizzle the dressing over the zucchini carpaccio, then if possible serve warm.

Time: 20 minutes
Difficulty: Easy

Nutrition facts per serving:
Calories: 90 kcal
Fat: 8 g
Protein: 4.2 g
Carbohydrates 2.1 g

Carrot Curry

Ingredients for 4 servings:
- 6 carrots
- 4 parsley roots
- 1 Spanish onion
- 7 Tbs (100 ml) vegetable broth
- 3 1/2 Tbs (50 ml) milk
- 1/2 c (100 ml) whipping cream
- 3 tsp curry paste
- Cilantro to garnish
- Oil
- Salt and pepper to season

Directions:
1. To prepare the vegetables, first peel and slice the Spanish onion. If the onion is very big, cut the slices in half so the pieces are bite size. Then either chop or slice the carrots. Do the same with the parsley roots.
2. Heat a pot with oil on the stove and first lightly braise the Spanish onion in it until it takes some color. Then add the remaining vegetables and sauté for 3 more minutes. Then add the vegetable broth, cream and milk and boil down for 15 minutes.
3. Add the curry powder and the curry paste and cook everything on medium for 5 more minutes. Season to taste with salt and pepper and garnish with the plucked cilantro.

Time: 30 minutes
Difficulty: Easy

Nutrition facts per serving:
Calories: 188 kcal
Fat: 11.8 g
Protein: 2.7 g
Carbohydrates 9.9 g

Kohlrabi Au Gratin

Ingredients for 4 servings:
- 1 lb (500 g) kohlrabi
- 3/4 c (100 g) shredded cheese
- 1/2 c (100 ml) whipping cream
- 3 Tbs (20 g) Parmesan
- 4 1/4 c (1 liter) vegetable broth
- ½ bunch of parsley
- ½ bunch of chives
- Nutmeg
- Salt and pepper to season

Directions:
1. Peel the kohlrabi and cut into bite size pieces. Cook in hot water or vegetable broth for about 5 -10 minutes.
2. Meanwhile prepare the sauce, mixing the cream and grated Parmesan and the chopped chives and parsley in a bowl. Scoop about 3/4 c (200 ml) of the warm vegetable broth into the bowl and mix in. Season with nutmeg and salt and pepper.
3. First spread a little of the sauce on the bottom. Then spread out the precooked kohlrabi. Pour in the rest of the sauce and top with the cheese. Bake in a preheated oven at 350°F (180°C) for 25 minutes and serve warm from the casserole or on plates.

Time: 30 minutes
Difficulty: Mean

Nutrition facts per serving:
Calories: 260 kcal
Fat: 17.1 g
Protein: 15 g
Carbohydrates 7.4 g

Scalloped Fennel

Ingredients for 4 servings:
- 4 bulbs of fennel
- 3 1/2 c (750 ml) vegetable broth
- 5 oz (150 g) mozzarella
- Olive oil
- Salt and pepper to season

Directions:
1. To prepare the bulbs of fennel, remove the stalk and leaves. Cook the remaining bulb in hot water with salt or vegetable broth for about 10 minutes. Then cut the fennel in half and add into a casserole dish. Season with salt and pepper.
2. Add a little of the vegetable broth and top the halves with the sliced mozzarella. Bake in a preheated oven at 400°F (200°C) for 10-15 minutes. Once the mozzarella is golden brown the food is done. Serve warm.

Time: 30 minutes
Difficulty: Easy

Nutrition facts per serving:
Calories: 200 kcal
Fat: 13.1 g
Protein: 12.6 g
Carbohydrates 6.6 g

Dinner Recipes

Parmesan-Crusted Celery Scallops

Ingredients for 4 servings:
- 1 celery root
- 2/3 c (50 g) coconut flakes
- 2 eggs
- Oil
- Salt and pepper to season

Directions:
1. Peel the celery root with a knife and slice about 3/4 inch (2 cm) thick.
2. Set out two plates for the breading. Whisk two eggs with a little salt and pepper on one. Pour the coconut flakes on the other. First coat both sides of the celery slices in egg, then in coconut flakes.
3. Heat a pan with oil and cook the celery scallops from both sides until golden brown. Cook on medium so the coconut flakes won't burn. Serve the celery scallops warm.

Time: 20 minutes
Difficulty: Easy

Nutrition facts per serving:
Calories: 190 kcal
Fat: 16.5 g
Protein: 5.9 g
Carbohydrates 3 g

Sage Omelet

Ingredients for 4 servings:
- 6 eggs
- 5 oz (150 g) king oyster mushrooms
- 20 sage leaves
- 1 onion
- Oil
- Salt and pepper to season

Directions:
1. Dice the onion and slice the king oyster mushrooms. First sauté the onions in a pan until they take color. Then add the king oyster mushrooms and sauté from both sides until golden brown.
2. Add the eggs, sage leaves and salt and pepper to a shaker and blend a little. Pour the mixture over the contents in the pan and bake in a preheated oven at 400°F (200°C) for 10-15 minutes.
3. Carefully move the omelet to a platter and cut into pizza slices, then serve warm.

Time: 25 minutes
Difficulty: Easy

Nutrition facts per serving:
Calories: 195 kcal
Fat: 14.5 g
Protein: 12.5 g
Carbohydrates 2 g

Parsnip Stir-Fry

Ingredients for 4 servings:
- 3 parsnips
- 2 kohlrabi
- 1 onion
- 3 tbs (40 g) butter
- 1 any frozen mixed herbs
- 2 Tbs parsley
- Salt and pepper to season

Directions:
1. First mix the butter, the mixed herbs and salt and pepper and refrigerate until solid.
2. Then peel the vegetables and cut into thin, bite size slices. Also peel the onion, cut in half and slice. In a pan melt the herb butter and first lightly braise the onions in it until translucent.
3. Next add the parsnips and kohlrabi and lightly braise over 10 minutes, stirring constantly. Then chop the parsley and add to the pan. Reduce the heat again and cook 5 more minutes.
4. Season to taste with salt and pepper before it is done cooking.

Time: 25 minutes
Difficulty: Easy

Nutrition facts per serving:
Calories: 105 kcal
Fat: 8.7 g
Protein: 2.2 g
Carbohydrates 4.4 g

Pumpkin-Mozzarella Casserole

Ingredients for 4 servings:
- 1 lb (500) squash
- 7 oz (200 g) mozzarella balls
- 3/4 oz (25 g) ginger
- 2 1/2 Tbs (20 g) pine nuts
- Oil
- Salt and pepper to season

Directions:
1. First cut the squash in half and use a spoon to remove the seeds. Cut the squash into quarters and place on a cookie sheet. Precook at 300°F (150°C) for about 25 minutes.
2. Meanwhile peel and thinly slice the ginger. When the cooking time is up, cut the squash into bite size pieces and place in a casserole dish brushed with olive oil. Add the mozzarella balls, pine nuts and ginger. Season with salt and pepper and carefully mix with a spoon.
3. Bake at 400°F (200°C) for 35 minutes.

Time: 45 minutes
Difficulty: Easy

Nutrition facts per serving:
Calories: 226 kcal
Fat: 17.7 g
Protein: 11.4 g
Carbohydrates 3.7 g

Stuffed Mushrooms

Ingredients for 4 servings:
- 8 large white mushrooms
- 3/4 c (20 g) dried mushrooms
- 3 Tbs (20 g) sun-dried tomatoes
- 1 red onion
- 1 Tbs parsley
- Oil
- Cayenne
- Salt

Directions:
1. Thinly coat two sheets of aluminum foil halfway with olive oil. Now carefully remove the stems from the white mushrooms and place four onto each sheet of aluminum foil.
2. For the stuffing, in a blender process the sun-dried tomatoes and mushrooms along with the stems from the white mushrooms and the red onions and parsley. Season with salt and cayenne pepper.
3. Divide over the white mushrooms, then cover the white mushrooms with the second sheet of aluminum foil. Bake at 350°F (180°C) for 15 minutes, then serve warm in the aluminum foil.

Time: 25 minutes
Difficulty: Easy

Nutrition facts per serving:
Calories: 74 kcal
Fat: 5.5 g
Protein: 3.2 g
Carbohydrates 1.9 g

Baked Asparagus

Ingredients for 4 servings:
- 1 lb (500 g) asparagus (white or green)
- 7 oz (200 g) feta
- 7 Tbs (100 ml) vegetable broth
- 4 green onions
- Oil
- Salt and pepper to season

Directions:
1. As a first step you should already set out the casserole dish for the asparagus.
2. You will now need the asparagus, will be added to the casserole dish once peeled (if white) and seasoned with salt and pepper.
3. Now thinly slice the green onions and sprinkle the asparagus with the green onions and parsley. Add the feta, which should be crumbled over it. Then sprinkle a little high quality oil over the mixture.
4. Bake for about half an hour, then enjoy a delicious meal.

Time: 35 minutes
Difficulty: Mean

Nutrition facts per serving:
Calories: 205 kcal
Fat: 14.6 g
Protein: 11.2 g
Carbohydrates 5.5 g

Vegetable Kebabs

Ingredients for 4 servings:
- 6 white mushrooms
- 6 shallots
- 3 1/2 oz (100 g) tofu
- Chili powder
- Sesame seeds
- Oil
- Salt and pepper to season

Directions:
1. First carefully roast the sesame seeds in the pan. Then mix the chili powder, sesame seeds and oil. Next chop the shallots and white mushrooms. You can also cut the tofu into cubes.
2. Now thread the tofu, shallots and mushrooms onto skewers, paying attention to variety. Then bake for max. eight minutes at medium heat. When done grilling, brush the kebabs with the chili paste and maybe also season the kebabs.

Time: 20 minutes
Difficulty: Easy

Nutrition facts per serving:
Calories: 114 kcal
Fat: 9.3 g
Protein: 4.8 g
Carbohydrates 2.2 g

Eggplant Lasagna

Ingredients for 4 servings:
- 1 large can of tomatoes
- 2 eggplants
- 2 carrots
- 1 onion
- 1 garlic clove
- 9 oz (250 g) tofu
- 1 1/3 c (150 g) shredded cheese
- 2 oz (50 g) Parmesan
- 1 pkg. frozen Italian herbs
- Garnish with basil
- Oregano
- Oil
- Salt and pepper to season

Directions:
1. First slice the eggplant and sauté until golden brown in a pan with oil.
2. Now cut the tofu into small pieces and add to the pan. Now cook the tofu with the Italian herbs. Add diced carrots, garlic and onion. Add the shredded cheese and the Parmesan for a very creamy sauce.
3. Now layer the sauce and sliced eggplant in the casserole dish. If you like cheese, you can add more cheese over the top.
4. This lasagna is a fruity and cheesy delight which will thrill all lasagna lovers.

Time: 40 minutes
Difficulty: Easy

Nutrition facts per serving:
Calories: 330 kcal
Fat: 21 g

Protein: 21.7 g
Carbohydrates 10.7 g

Stuffed Peppers

Ingredients for 4 servings:
- 4 orange bell peppers
- 1/4 lb (100 g) cocktail tomatoes
- 2 oz (50 g) Parmesan
- 1 green chili pepper
- 3 Tbs (50 g) crème fraîche
- 1 tsp Tabasco
- Fresh herbs of your choice
- Oil
- Salt and pepper to season

Directions:
1. First cut the bell peppers in half and remove the white skin and seeds.
2. For the stuffing cut the chili and quarter the tomatoes. In a bowl, mix both ingredients with herbs and Tabasco and crème fraîche. If desired, season to taste with salt and pepper.
3. Now place the bell pepper halves on a cookie sheet and use equal amounts of the contents of the bowl as the stuffing. Sprinkle with Parmesan and in a preheated oven at 350°F (175°C) for 25 minutes.

Time: 40 minutes
Difficulty: Easy

Nutrition facts per serving:
Calories: 225 kcal
Fat: 15.8 g
Protein: 11.6 g
Carbohydrates 7.6 g

Cauliflower Casserole

Ingredients for 4 servings:
- 1 head of cauliflower
- 1 onion
- 1 egg
- 2/3 c (150 g) yogurt
- 1/2 c (100 g) sour cream
- 3/4 c (100 g) shredded cheese
- 3 Tbs (25 g) pine nuts
- 3 Tbs (25 g) sunflower seeds
- 2 Tbs parsley
- 1 Tbs vegetable broth
- 1 dash nutmeg
- Salt and pepper to season

Directions:
1. Before cooking you should first set out the casserole dish. Then cut the cauliflower into little florets, the sunflower seeds and pine nuts should be roasted.
2. Dice the onion, sauté in the pan, then mix with vegetable broth, yogurt, egg and sour cream. Add the shredded cheese, then add the different seeds to this mixture.
3. Brush the casserole dish with oil and add the cauliflower. Top with the mixture with the seeds and if you like your casserole with lots of cheese you can add another serving of shredded cheese.
4. Preheat the oven to 400°F (200°C) and after max. 40 minutes you will have a casserole to impress any vegetable lover.

Time: 45 minutes
Difficulty: Easy

Nutrition facts per serving:
Calories: 288 kcal
Fat: 20.3 g

Protein: 15.6 g
Carbohydrates 8.5 g

Snacks

Pepper Snack

Ingredients for 4 servings:
- 1 c (200 g) pimento
- Olive oil
- Salt

Directions:
1. Heat a pan with a little oil on the stove and sautée the pimento from all sides until golden brown.
2. Drain on paper towel and sprinkle with a pinch salt before serving.

Time: 10 minutes
Difficulty: Easy

Nutrition facts per serving:
Calories: 56.1 kcal
Fat: 5.1 g
Protein: 0.6 g
Carbohydrates 1.4 g

Spicy Kale Chips

Ingredients for 4 servings:
- 1 lb (500 g) fresh kale
- Chili powder
- Salt

Directions:
1. Wash the kale leaves and dry with a salad spinner. Then cut into bite size pieces and arrange on a cookie sheet lined with parchment paper. Bake in a preheated oven at 250°f (125°c) for 10 minutes until crisp.
2. Before serving, sprinkle with salt and chili powder in a bowl and stir well to evenly coat the kale chips.

Time: 20 minutes
Difficulty: Mean

Nutrition facts per serving:
Calories: 22.6 kcal
Fat: 0.7 g
Protein: 2.3 g
Carbohydrates 1.6 g

Dolmades

Ingredients for 4 servings:
- 12 grape leaves
- 6 marinated bell peppers
- 1/4 c (25 g) sun-dried tomatoes
- 2 oz (50 g) Parmesan
- 2 1/2 Tbs (20 g) pine nuts
- 6 olives
- Oil
- Salt and pepper to season

Directions:
1. For the stuffing first add the marinated bell pepper with the pine nuts, olives and sun-dried tomatoes into a blender and blend. Then add the grated Parmesan and also blend to make everything into a mixture. Then season with salt and pepper if desired.
2. Lay out the ready to eat grape leaves and divide the stuffing equally over the leaves. Then make into little roll-ups. These can be eaten cold or heat in a pan for 1 minute each side.

Time: 30 minutes
Difficulty: Easy

Nutrition facts per serving:
Calories: 153 kcal
Fat: 11.5 g
Protein: 7.2 g
Carbohydrates 3.6 g

Carrot Patties

Ingredients for 4 servings:
- 1/2 lb (250 g) carrots
- 1 egg
- ½ bunch of parsley
- 6 mint leaves
- 2 Tbs ground almonds
- Oil
- Salt and pepper to season

Directions:
1. In a first step, shred the peeled carrots. Add the flour and egg to the shredded carrots and mix well. Add the chopped parsley and you are ready to cook everything into delicious carrot patties.
2. For a delicious bonus, garnish with ground almonds and mint leaves.

Time: 30 minutes
Difficulty: Easy

Nutrition facts per serving:
Calories: 120 kcal
Fat: 8 g
Protein: 4.1 g
Carbohydrates 6.8 g

Chicory Boats

Ingredients for 4 servings:
- 1 chicory
- 2/3 c (150 g) chive & onion cream cheese
- 1 c (25 g) dried mushrooms
- 3 Tbs (25 g) chopped walnuts
- Curry powder
- Salt and pepper to season

Directions:
1. Trim the woody ends from the chicory, remove the individual leaves and place on a platter.
2. For the stuffing, in a bowl mix the cream cheese, chopped walnuts and dried mushrooms. Then season to taste with curry powder, salt and pepper.
3. Divide the stuffing equally over the lettuce and either serve promptly or refrigerate.

Time: 15 minutes
Difficulty: Easy

Nutrition facts per serving:
Calories: 200 kcal
Fat: 15.6 g
Protein: 10.4 g
Carbohydrates 2.4 g

Pumpkin Chips with Parmesan

Ingredients for 4 servings:
- 2/3 lb (300 g) squash
- 2 oz (50 g) Parmesan
- Oil
- Salt and pepper to season

Directions:
1. Thinly slice the squash flesh and arrange on a cookie sheet lined with parchment paper. Bake the squash chips in a preheated oven at 350°F (175°C) for 25 minutes.
2. 10 minutes before done baking, sprinkle the squash with Parmesan and finish baking. Allow to cool, then serve in a bowl.

Time: 40 minutes
Difficulty: Easy

Nutrition facts per serving:
Calories: 78 kcal
Fat: 6.2 g
Protein: 5.1 g
Carbohydrates 2.2 g

Vegetarian Patty

Ingredients for 4 servings:
- 4 1/2 oz (125 g) feta
- 1/3 lb (150 g) broccoli
- 2 1/2 oz (75 g) zucchini
- 2 carrots
- 1 onion
- 1 garlic clove
- Oil
- Salt and pepper to season

Directions:
1. Use a food processor for the first step to make it easier. It can be used to chop the onion, carrots, zucchini, broccoli and the garlic clove and process into a mixture.
2. Mix well with the feta, salt and pepper, roll the mixture into little balls and cook well in a pan. The mixture can be rolled into balls or a nice size patty, then sautée in oil make a delicious dish even meat eaters will love.

Time: 30 minutes
Difficulty: Easy

Nutrition facts per serving:
Calories: 155 kcal
Fat: 11.1 g
Protein: 7.5 g
Carbohydrates 5.1 g

Stuffed Tomatoes

Ingredients for 4 servings:
- 4 beefsteak tomatoes
- 1 eggplant
- 1 mozzarella
- Salt and pepper to season

Directions:
1. In a first step cut the wash tomatoes in half and carefully scoop out with a spoon. Do the same with the eggplant.
2. Drop the flesh of the tomatoes and eggplant into a bowl and mix with salt and pepper. Thinly slice the mozzarella.
3. Now stuff the tomatoes with the mixture and top each tomato with a slice of mozzarella.
4. Bake the tomatoes in the oven until the cheese is golden brown.
5. Serve as a little snack or as a delicious side with other dishes, these tomatoes are always a hit.

Time: 30 minutes
Difficulty: Easy

Nutrition facts per serving:
Calories: 163 kcal
Fat: 12.5 g
Protein: 8.3 g
Carbohydrates 2.8 g

Baked Chèvre

Ingredients for 4 servings:
- 4 slices chèvre
- Balsamic vinegar
- Mustard
- Honey
- Salt and pepper to season

Directions:
1. Arrange the sliced cheese in a casserole dish.
2. Now mix vinegar, mustard, pepper, salt and honey and spread over the cheese.
3. The chèvre doesn't take long to bake, max. 4 minutes will be enough.
4. The cheese tastes great on a fresh slice of cloud bread or enjoy by itself for a cheesy treat.

Time: 20 minutes
Difficulty: Easy

Nutrition facts per serving:
Calories: 450 kcal
Fat: 31.8 g
Protein: 31.1 g
Carbohydrates 4.1 g

Tofu Patties

Ingredients for 4 servings:
- 10 oz (300 g) tofu
- 2/3 c (75 g) shredded cheese
- 1 egg
- 1 red onion
- 1 green chili pepper
- 2 Tbs parsley
- Oil
- Salt and pepper to season

Directions:
1. First prepare the tofu, which is best diced.
2. For the patty mixture now chop the onions and chili. Chop the parsley. Then blend everything with the egg and cheese into a mixture. If you'd like, you can now add salt and pepper.
3. Heat the oil in a pan, shape the tofu patties and sautée in the pan.
4. These patties make a great light snack that won't leave you hungry. As a little something extra, make a light dip.

Time: 25 minutes
Difficulty: Mean

Nutrition facts per serving:
Calories: 174 kcal
Fat: 13.9 g
Protein: 12.2 g
Carbohydrates 1.8 g

CONCLUSION

Combining vegetarian and vegan cooking with the principles of low carb truly enriches your diet instead of restricting it even more. After all, a meatless diet doesn't automatically mean physical fitness and weight loss. If the meat is simply replaced with carbs, the opposite can happen and you will actually gain weight.

This cookbook is a convenient manual for vegetarians and vegans for a healthy, balanced diet and finally seeing the desired success when you step on the scale. From quick snacks to dinners the entire family and guests will enjoy, this cookbook features recipes for every meal. Combining low carb and a meatless diet is therefore definitely even worth a 14 day journey for meat lovers.

Yours truly,

Mathias Müller

AUTHOR

Low carb, full flavor - in this wonderful cookbook Mathias Müller explains over 50 basic recipes in detail. Müller's clear-cut, passionate writing not only inspire novices to follow their intuition in the kitchen and understand the essence of a recipe: 'Honestly, good food is nothing more than good ingredients prepared simply'. And the large chapter on meat and fish entrées also includes vegetarian versions. There are lots of delicious and easy recipes for a healthy diet to cook for any meal.

'HEALTHY LIVING' is Müller's philosophy which comes to life in every line of this new edition of the classic "50 Vegetarian and Vegan Recipes for Successful Weight Loss in Just 2 Weeks". Müller has published various bestsellers:

"Low Carb Recipes - 50 Lunch Recipes for Successful Weight Loss in Just 2 Weeks"

"Low Carb Recipes – 50 Dinners for Permanent Weight Loss Success"

"Low Carb Recipes - 50 Vegetarian and Vegan Recipes for Successful Weight Loss in Just 2 Weeks"

"Low Carb Recipes – 14-Day Plan with Delicious Recipes for Permanent Weight Loss at Home and on the Road"

"Low Carb Recipes - 100 Low Carb breakfast recipes for successful weight loss in 2 weeks"

"Low Carb Recipes - 100 Low Carb Desserts for Successful Weight Loss in 2 Weeks"

"Low Carb Recipes – 300 Low Carb Recipes for Permanent Weight Loss Success"